*Welcome to your Walking Stick Press guided
journal. Within these pages you'll find:*

*

instruction to guide you

*

writing prompts to help you explore

*

blank pages to record your responses to the
prompts—to map your path

*

quotes to inspire, provoke, and refresh you

*

*Along the way, feel free to jot in the margins,
add your own quotes,
let writing take you down a trail you didn't expect.
Enjoy the journey.*

*

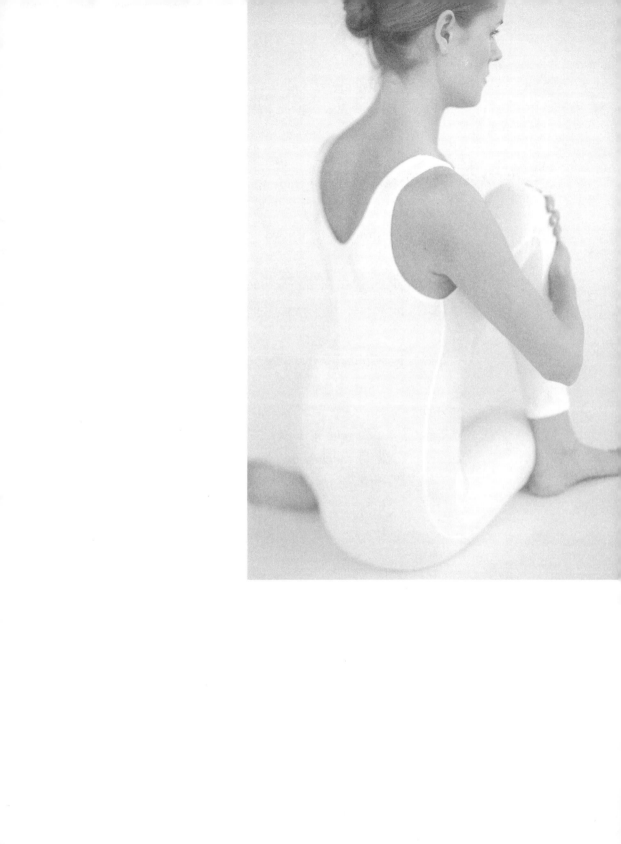

my yoga journal

guided reflections through writing

VICTORIA MORAN

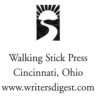

Walking Stick Press
Cincinnati, Ohio
www.writersdigest.com

Visit our Web site at www.writersdigest.com for information on more resources for writers.

To receive a free weekly E-mail newsletter delivering tips and updates about writing and about Writer's Digest products, register directly at our Web site at http://newsletters.fwpublications.com.

06 05 04 03 02   5 4 3 2 1

Library of Congress Cataloging-in-Publication Data
Moran, Victoria
    My yoga journal: guided reflections through writing/Victoria Moran.
        p. cm.
    Includes bibliographical references.
    ISBN 1-58297-099-8 (alk.paper)
        1. Yoga, Hatha. 2. Diaries–Authorship–Problems, exercises, etc. I. Title.

RA781.7.M65 2002
613.7'046–dc21   2001045348
                                                         CIP

Edited by Jack Heffron and Donya Dickerson
Interior designed by Brian Roeth
Cover designed by Stephanie Strang
Cover photography by Photodisc
Production coordinated by Kristen Heller

dedication

To my teachers past and present:
    Mildred Jensen,
    Stella Cherfas,
    Sushila Peterson,
    Valda Anderson,
    GuruParwaz Khalsa,
    Panchali Null

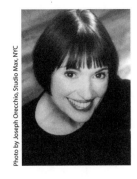

Victoria Moran, an author and national speaker, has been a student of yoga for over thirty years and a journal-keeper for nearly twenty. Her other books include:

* *Body Confident: A Guided Journal for Losing Weight and Feeling Great,* another guided journal in this series
* *Lit from Within: Tending Your Soul for Lifelong Beauty*
* *Creating a Charmed Life: Sensible, Spiritual Secrets Every Busy Woman Should Know*
* *Shelter for the Spirit: Create Your Own Haven in a Hectic World*
* *Love Yourself Thin: The Revolutionary Spiritual Approach to Weight Loss*

Her articles have appeared in publications including *Yoga Journal, Personal Journaling, Vegetarian Times, Ladies' Home Journal,* and *Woman's Day.*

To learn more about Victoria's work or to book her as a speaker for your organization, visit her Web site: www.victoriamoran.com.

about the **author**

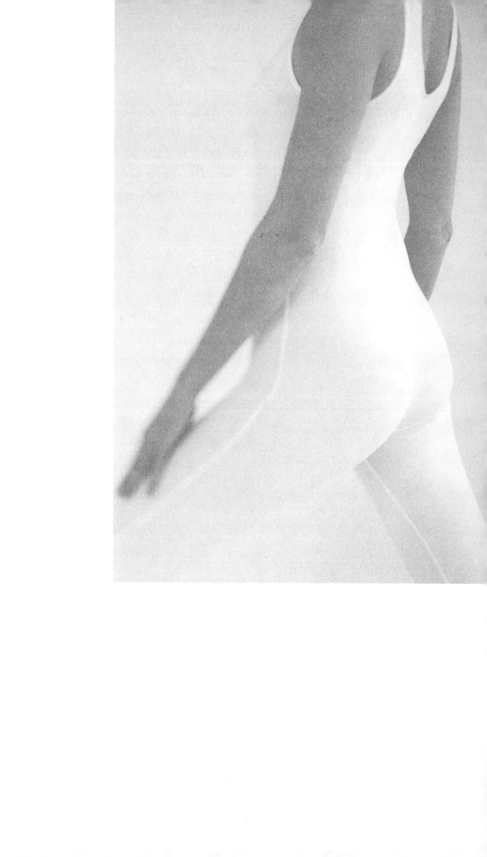

table of contents

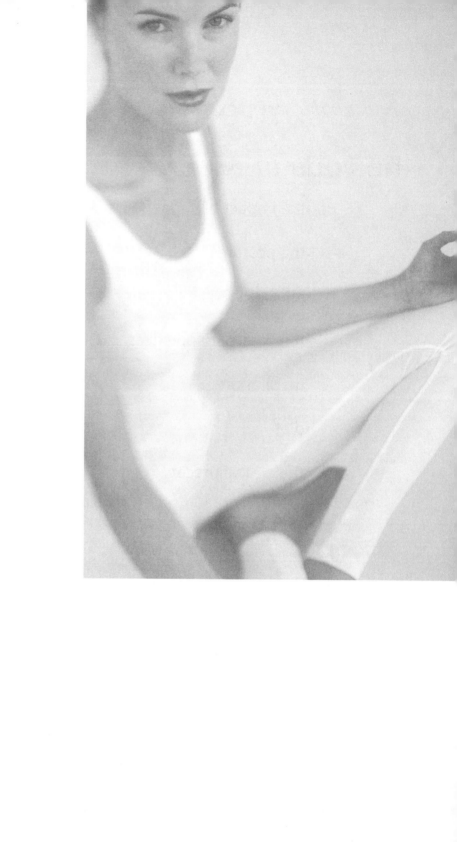

how to use this book:

the yoga of the pen

Most of us enroll in yoga class expecting to engage in stretching and strengthening movements that, over time, will make us look and feel better. Maybe we want to lose some weight or have a firmer, more toned body. Or we have stressful jobs and want to work off some of the tension we bring home from them. Or we feel guilty about not exercising and figure we ought to do something physical.

But joining a gym or taking up jogging would accomplish these goals. We who are drawn to yoga tend to be looking for something more, either consciously or at some deeper level. We may be seeking more meaning in our lives. Or greater self-control. Or to know ourselves better. These are among the promises of yoga. And keeping this journal as a companion to your practice will further ensure that these promises—and everything else you hope for from your yoga practice—will be fulfilled.

Since you have purchased this journal, we can assume that you are taking yoga classes, that you used to take class and you now practice on your own, or that you're teaching yourself yoga through a book or video. Therefore, *My Yoga Journal* is not an instruction manual. It is, instead, a tool for enriching the practice you already have. Its chapters are arranged to mirror the traditional order of a full yoga session, treating postures, relaxation, breathing practices, and meditation in turn. The final two chapters address yoga's dietary principles and ethical teachings—popular topics for the after-class discussions many yoga teachers offer their students.

This book will aid your progress in two important ways. First, the boxes entitled "My Yoga Path" are for you to write about your hatha yoga practice itself. You can write about the *asana* (posture) that's your current favorite, how it makes you feel, and how your body is responding to the progress you're making on it. Or you can write about a troublesome posture, one that your body doesn't seem to take to naturally or that you just don't seem to "get."

As you make notes about the postures, you'll find that each one becomes a metaphor for other areas of your life. If you're stiff in the full forward bend, for example, you may want to respond with "loosening up" your attitude a little in your day-to-day life. You might confront a tendency toward shyness or low self-esteem by using your mind to help you really *inhabit* the confidence-building lion pose (*simhasana*). If you can feel like king of the jungle, it follows that you can

my yoga path

How did my yoga practice go today?

Sun salute felt better — I've got the order memorized finally. Still can't do shoulderstand — hurts my neck — had to do legs-up-the-wall alternative. Wanted to push myself and ignore the pain but did the right thing.

also feel capable of speaking for a group or asking for a raise.

You might use some "My Yoga Path" boxes to note how you're doing with *pranayama* (the yogic breathing exercises), to track your experience with meditation, or simply to congratulate yourself for showing up to do your yoga practice.

The bulk of these pages, however, are for writing what comes to you as you consider your life experience as a spiritual being and a student of yoga. The prompts provided at the end of each chapter are like the energy from another car's battery that can jump-start yours. They're an impetus, a nudge. They'll get you started. Once they do, you're on your own. As you write, never force yourself to "stay with the subject." Journal-writing is a nonlinear process of self-discovery, much like yoga itself. You could call it "the yoga of the pen."

If you're a writer by nature or if you're accustomed to keeping a diary or journal, you might use the prompts simply as starting points for getting what's on your mind onto paper. If journaling is new to you, however, and you've never thought of writing as a way to spend leisure time, the prompts can mentor you through the process. They can even help you focus your thoughts on a topic that may have layers underneath.

For example, a prompt may ask you to write about how regular you are with your yoga practice. You might write that you've had a hard time doing your morning practice lately because you've been hitting the snooze button on your alarm clock—repeatedly. As you continue, you may find yourself writing that you've had trouble sleeping ever since your job transfer. This connection may lead you to write a page or more about your new responsibilities at work and how you can make them more manageable.

"Hey, I thought this was supposed to be a yoga journal." Precisely. Yoga is about improving your life. Every time you write something on these pages that does that, or that makes you feel better about your life the way it is, then you're using this journal just the way you're supposed to.

Like your yoga practice, your writing practice is yours alone. Choose the prompts that interest you, and skip the others without regret. You may want to go back to them later (even after you finish this journal and you've gone on to another one) or to record your extraordinary ideas in an ordinary notebook. Some of the prompts in *My Yoga Journal* have more than one question or suggestion. They're here to spur your thinking, but you needn't feel obligated to address all of them unless you want to.

It's also up to you to decide when to write and for how long. You may want to include journaling in your daily period of quiet time when you do yoga postures and meditation. Most people do journal-writing in the early morning, but for others nighttime is best. You may even carve out writing time during part of your lunch hour.

If writing every day is more of a commitment than you want to make, coordinate your use of this journal with your yoga class schedule. Get to class early, and write in the practice room as the other students gather. Or make an appointment with yourself to go to a café after class, and write while you sip your juice or tea.

Just as you come to know your physical strengths and limitations by attempting more challenging postures, you come to know your inner self through writing. And just as your physical capabilities will sometimes astonish you as you continue with yoga ("I stood on my head. Me! This is incredible."), the words you write may surprise you, too.

This self-discovery through writing comes from the uncanny link between the hand and the brain and, as you continue journaling, between the act of writing and the human psyche. You will find yourself writing what you know as you record events and work through feelings; and—amazingly—you will find yourself writing what you didn't realize you already knew. You'll be tapping inner wisdom and intuitive depths that most of us disregard in our busy lives.

The definition of the Sanskrit word *yoga* is *union*: union with the self, union with all people and all of nature, and ultimately union with the divine. When yoga joins with journal-writing, you have a winning combination. Of course, yoga is not about winning. It is about *being*: being fully conscious, fully aware, fully alive. May what you read in this book—and most of all what you write in it—add to the fullness of your life.

my life priorities

Make a hierarchical list of the important components in your life (i.e., your family, job, house, etc.). Where does yoga fit into this list? How could it move higher on your list? Check in on a monthly basis to see how your priorities have moved around.

1. _____

   _____

2. _____

   _____

3. _____

   _____

4. _____

   _____

5. _____

   _____

6. _____

   _____

7. _____

   _____

8. _____

   _____

9. _____

   _____

10. _____

    _____

| my time |

Take a week to observe the various activities in your life. In the boxes below, write the hours you are spending on each activity. Are there places in your day where you can make more time for yoga?

	DAY 1	DAY 2	DAY 3	DAY 4	DAY 5	DAY 6	DAY 7
family time							
work, school							
errands, chores							
driving time							
yoga							
meditation							
church, volunteering, meetings							
television							
food preparation, meals							
recreation, creative pursuits							

check in

At the end of every section of blank pages, you'll find a Check In page. Use this page for general explorations of yourself and your yoga practice. For this first Check In, write what you'd like to get out of this book.

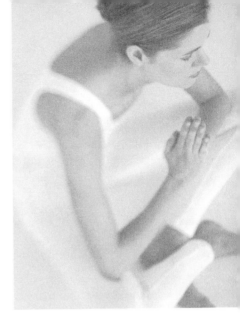

chapter one

the impact
of yoga

Attending your first yoga class can be like having your first child: Until you do it, you have no idea how profoundly this step will change your life.

I first looked into yoga at the age of seventeen. This time-honored practice was enjoying a resurgence in the West at that time, as it is now. Then it was because the Beatles were meditating. And air travel had become cheap enough for an assortment of swamis—some holy and sincere, others wholly insincere—to make their way to America.

My earliest yoga classes were held on the basketball court of a midwestern YWCA. I started primarily because I'd heard yoga could make me thin and secondarily because I'd heard it could make me wise. What struck me initially was that, unlike in other exercise classes, the students weren't competing with one another. For much of the class, we were actually supposed to keep our eyes closed.

I also noted that yoga had a unique attitude of gentleness that seemed to echo the graceful, fluid movements of the postures themselves. In classical hatha yoga and in most of the variations it's spawned, the movements are slow and usually held for a time, an act of cooperation of earth and space with the will and the skill of the student.

Yoga also differs from many other exercise forms in that the teacher is not there to issue commands but to impart wisdom. My first instructor didn't talk a lot, but what she said stuck: "Don't compare yourself with other people; think of our class as one body so each person's progress can belong to all of us. . . . If it hurts, back off: In yoga we say, 'If pain, no gain'. . . . Don't force changes on your body or your life; allow positive changes to happen. . . . "

In time I started seeing those changes—first in my body (it was stronger, firmer, more flexible) and then in my world view. Yoga's messages—relax, let go, breathe, remember who you are—began to replace society's messages of push, shove, get ahead, look out for number one, and even, "Do something about those awful thighs." The yogic transformation had begun in me, as you have probably seen it develop in you, laying a foundation of attitudes that work better than the old ones did.

Many of these attitudes are rooted in nature. The bulk of the classic postures are named for animals and seek to emulate their movements and borrow from their strengths. The breathing practices make us appreciate clean air. The yogic diet makes us delight in natural foods. Even the ideal attire for yoga practice is loose clothing made of natural fibers—soft cotton, organic if you can get it, that lets your pores breathe and assists in the detoxification that the *asanas* precipitate.

As you practice in the coming weeks, and as you write about your practice and about your life in this journal, watch for the ways yoga impacts your life. Be aware of the subtle changes—not just in the way your clothes fit but in the way your days work.

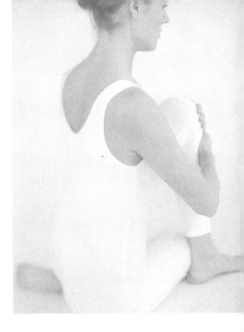

writing prompts

Let these suggestions spur your writing.
Don't feel the need to respond to all of them;
just write about the ones that speak to your heart.

1. Make a list of all the benefits you know of that yoga is purported to produce. Put a check mark after each one on which your yoga practice is already delivering.

2. What initially drew you to yoga? How is your practice delivering on that original attraction? How could it provide more of what you're looking for?

3. Yoga is about balance, about finding serenity in the midst of what we like and what we don't. What makes you happiest about your yoga practice? What do you find frustrating? What are you learning from both those parts that are appealing and those that are discouraging?

4. Are you treating yourself as gently as yoga suggests? How do you reconcile this gentleness with striving for progress in your practice? How do you interpret "progress" as a yoga student?

5. In a world of image makers and putting a "spin" on facts, yoga takes a stand for the authentic and the eternal. Write about who you are deep inside where your public visage doesn't go. How is yoga helping you get closer to this true self of yours?

6. What comes to mind when you think of a yogic way of life? What aspects of it would you like to incorporate into your life? How best can you do this?

my yoga calendar

For the next thirty days, record how long you spend each day doing yoga. It's okay if you leave days blank. At the end of the month, reflect on the amount of time you have for yoga. Are you surprised? If you want, make a copy of this chart before you fill it in and make a new chart when you feel the amount you do yoga has changed.

SUNDAY	MONDAY	TUESDAY	WEDNESDAY	THURSDAY	FRIDAY	SATURDAY

*Those who forget how
to blossom are evidently
branching off in the
wrong direction.*

LEO VROMAN

my yoga path

How did my yoga practice go today?

my yoga path

How did my yoga practice go today?

Never be entirely idle;
but either be reading, or
writing, or praying, or
meditating, or endeavoring
something for the public
good.

SANSKRIT PROVERB

Yoga is not a religion. It is crystallized truth.

SELVARAJAN YESUDIAN AND
ELISABETH HATCH

my yoga path

How did my yoga practice go today?

my yoga path

How did my yoga practice go today?

*Looking through the eyes of
the divine nature you see . . .
the creator within the creation, and it is a wonderful,
wonderful world!*

PEACE PILGRIM

my yoga path

How did my yoga practice go today?

my yoga path

How did my yoga practice go today?

One must live the way one thinks or end up thinking the way one has lived.

PAUL BOURGET

my yoga path

How did my yoga practice go today?

| check in |

Use this page for general explorations of yourself and your yoga practice.

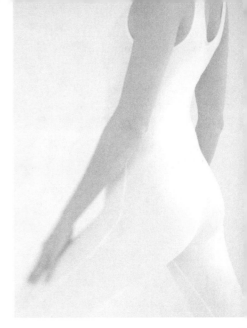

chapter two

the
postures

When you discovered yoga, did you see it as a wonderful adjunct to your already active life? Or were you a confirmed nonexerciser who was delighted to find a way to get fit that wouldn't demand more than you could give? One of the gifts of yoga is its ability to span the spectrum of fitness levels. At one end are highly skilled yogis who equal or surpass any professional athlete in terms of strength, stamina, and flexibility. At the other are beginners who may not be in good enough shape for aerobics classes or jogging but who, with their doctor's okay, can enroll in a basic yoga course and make rapid progress toward a healthier body.

There are a variety of schools of yoga, all evolved from the same ancient roots, to meet every practitioner's needs. You might be studying:

Integral Yoga, classic postures performed slowly, held in time and space, and integrated with breath, chanting, relaxation, and meditation;

Iyengar Yoga, a precision practice named for its founder; includes many standing postures and uses various yoga "props" to assist progress and prevent injury;

Bikram Yoga, another founder-named system known

for a systematic posture routine practiced in a hot room to encourage sweating and elimination of toxins;

Kundalini Yoga, an athletic form designed to challenge the body and awaken latent spiritual energies;

Ashtanga Yoga, a series of powerful postures done in one continuous movement with a strong tie to the breath;

Kripalu Yoga, a slow, gentle dancelike form that progresses gradually to more challenging movements.

Whether you study one of these popular types or some other variation, all yoga postures—called asanas—are designed to both tone and relax the musculature. Many poses are, in fact, designed to stretch one part of the body while simultaneously strengthening another. *Asana* practice also lubricates joints, gently massages internal organs, and improves circulation. In addition, yoga philosophy teaches that the subtle life force called *prana*, the energy that permeates all living things, is freed up by means of the postures, thus improving both physical and mental health.

The definition of the Sanskrit word *asana* is "steady, relaxed pose," and the intent is to perform each posture in a steady, relaxed way, at the balance point of effort and ease. Moreover, in yoga, the mind and the breath are as involved with the proper execution of *asanas* as are the muscles and joints. This involvement of the mind is the link uniting the various forms of yoga offered in the West today.

Guidelines essential for enjoying the *asanas*, advancing your practice, and reaping its benefits include:

＊ Practice in a warm, pleasant area. If candles or incense would make your space feel more "yogic," include them. Use a mat appropriate to the style of yoga you practice: i.e., a thinner "sticky mat" for Iyengar or Bikram with their many standing postures, a folded quilt or thicker mat for Integral Yoga that includes more floor work.

* Early morning is the recommended time for practice. If this is not feasible, practice when you can but at the same time each day if possible. Wait at least one hour after a snack or three hours after a meal.

* Because yoga is about order and balance in mind and body, practice postures in the order in which you do them in class, even if you're only performing a few of them. This order is not arbitrary: It was developed by the yogis who perfected the system you're working with to channel just the right amount of *prana* through your body and brain. This way you'll finish energized and relaxed, not wired and exhausted.

* Practice every day, if only for a few minutes. When you do need to miss a day or more, accept that and start back as soon as you can. One abbreviated routine for hurried mornings is: (1) sun salutation (*surya namaskar*), (2) shoulderstand (*sarvangasana*), (3) a few rounds of alternate nostril breathing (*nadi suddhi*), and (4) a brief relaxation in the corpse pose (*savasana*).

Remember that yoga is a process, not a competition, even with yourself. Give each posture your best, but never strain to achieve a position. With diligent practice, you'll come closer every day to performing the posture as the masters envisioned it.

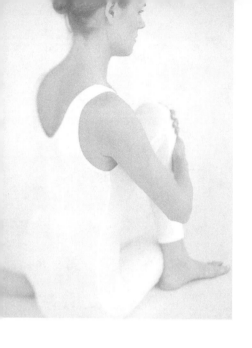

writing prompts

Let these suggestions spur your writing.
Don't feel the need to respond to all of them;
just write about the ones that speak to your heart.

1. Think about your attitude toward your body and physical activity in general. Do you consider yourself athletic? Graceful? Out of shape? How does yoga fit into your picture of yourself as a physical being?

2. List the physical changes that you observe in yourself from practicing yoga. Your list might note:
   * sleeping more soundly
   * climbing stairs with less effort
   * clearer skin
   * stopped telling toddler he's too heavy to pick up

3. Do some fantasy writing about your dream spot for practicing yoga. Maybe it's the patio of a beach house overlooking the Pacific or a large, spare studio with polished oak floors, gracious skylights, and Indian sitar music piped in. Describe your ideal place. Picture yourself there.

4. Now do some reality writing about the place where you actually practice. What can you do to make it more inviting? Make a realistic wish list for yourself.

5. Visualize your practice one year from now. What will you be doing that you aren't doing today? How will your body have changed? How about five years from now? Write this down.

my yoga practice

Use this chart to observe your own practice. In column one, write how you practice yoga now. Be honest and try not to judge yourself—simply observe. Column two is a place to describe your ideal practice, when and how you would practice yoga in the best of all possible worlds. For column three, write what is a possible practice for you—something realistic that falls between columns one and two.

	MY PRACTICE NOW	MY IDEAL PRACTICE	MY REALISTIC GOALS
number of days each week			
minutes per session			
time of day			
place			

*The posture of yoga is steady
and easy. It is realized by
relaxing one's effort and
resting like the cosmic serpent
on the waters of infinity.*

THE YOGA SUTRAS OF PATANJALI

my yoga path

How did my yoga practice go today?

my yoga path

How did my yoga practice go today?

Yoga has been practiced for thousands of years by millions of body types, and the Universe loves us all.

PANCHALI NULL,
YOGA PLUS INTERNATIONAL

my yoga path

How did my yoga practice go today?

Asanas . . . form the first stage of Hatha Yoga. One should practice asanas that make one firm, free of diseases, and light of limb.

HATHA YOGA PRADIPIKA

my yoga path

How did my yoga practice go today?

my yoga path

How did my yoga practice go today?

Good men spiritualize their bodies; bad men incarnate their souls.

BENJAMIN WHICHCOTE

*The Sun Salute (*Surya Namaskar*) is a complete Ayurvedic exercise that simultaneously integrates the whole physiology—mind, body, and breath.*

DEEPAK CHOPRA, M.D.,
*PERFECT HEALTH: THE
COMPLETE MIND/BODY GUIDE*

my yoga path

How did my yoga practice go today?

*My awareness of my body
is different than it used to
be . . . but it's not purely a
physical thing. [Yoga] also
leads you to a whole way of
approaching impulse and
trying to develop the observer,
which is a huge part of
performing—finding that
balance between letting go
and control, awareness and
abandon.*

WILLEM DAFOE

my yoga path

How did my yoga practice go today?

| check in |

Use this page for general explorations of yourself and your yoga practice.

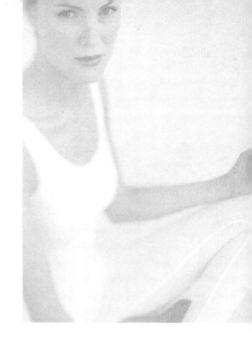

chapter three

relaxation

Did you ever think life would get so good that you'd do a form of exercise that has relaxation built in? Yoga is unique in the world of exercise in recognizing that relaxation is essential to reaping the benefits of activity. In fact, the relaxation position—corpse pose or *savasana,* lying on the back, feet comfortably apart, arms at the sides at the most comfortable place—is itself one of the *asanas.* Most yoga classes feature intermittent periods of *savasana* that help students relax their bodies and allow the effects of the previous movements to settle in.

In addition to *savasana,* many classes and full-length home practice sessions end with *yoga nidra.* This translates as "yogic sleep," although the aim is not to fall asleep but to enter a state of profound physical and mental rest. This is usually done while lying on a mat in *savasana,* covered with a blanket if you need it, since the body temperature tends to drop during this process. Give the suggestion to relax to each part of your body in turn, from your toes to your head. You can also do this by first tensing and then releasing the muscles of your feet, legs, buttocks, abdomen, etc. This tensing can enable the relaxation to be deeper and more penetrating.

With experience in relaxing at will—both brief relaxations throughout your practice time and intensive relaxation at the end—you will find that you can relax more easily when you need to at other times in your life. Yoga students who have been practicing relaxation for a while find they have less trouble falling asleep at night because the distance from "yogic sleep" to actual sleep is very short.

Being able to tap into this relaxed state during the day—even momentarily, without lying down or closing your eyes—is a vital component of yoga's anti-tension triple threat: relaxation, breath control, and meditation. Each of these three practices prepares the body and mind for the next one, just as *asanas* prepare the body and mind for relaxation.

With our Western penchant for action, beginners sometimes find relaxation practice boring or superfluous. Trust the wisdom of yoga tradition on this one. Relaxation is the flip side of exertion and is essential for maintaining balance. It is an introduction to quiet. It pays homage to your body for a job well done, and it can be the first phase in coming to know your true self.

writing prompts

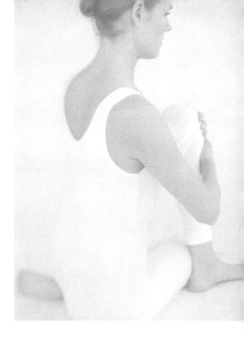

Let these suggestions spur your writing.
Don't feel the need to respond to all of them;
just write about the ones that speak to your heart.

1. Coming as we do from a culture based on striving and succeeding, how do you feel about being told to relax? Do you believe it has value or that it's a waste of time? Has yoga helped you become more relaxed?

2. Science is now telling us that most Westerners are sleep-deprived, contributing to weight problems, hypertension, diabetes, and accelerated aging. Assess your sleep life on paper. How much do you sleep? How well? How might you use yoga relaxation and other yogic practices to help you sleep soundly every night?

3. Write about (or draw if you'd like) some relaxing images: a backyard hammock, a still lake, a seaside sunset. Write what it feels like to be there, even if only in your imagination.

4. List the simple pleasures that help you relax. A good meal? A stroll in the park? An intimate conversation with the person you love most? How can you get more of these relaxing moments into your day?

my lifestyle

Your "lifestyle coach" has written you a letter of advice telling you to slow down.
Write that letter.

Dear _____ ,

Sincerely,
Your lifestyle coach

my yoga path

How did my yoga practice go today?

*Nothing gives rest but the
sincere search for truth.*

BLAISE PASCAL

*The world is imprisoned in
its own activity, except when
actions are performed as
worship of God.*

THE BHAGAVAD GITA

my yoga path

How did my yoga practice go today?

my yoga path

How did my yoga practice go today?

Do not mistake laziness for relaxation. The lazy man is inactive . . . full of lethargy and inertia. Whereas a man who practices relaxation . . . has vigor, strength, vitality, and endurance.

SWAMI SIVANANDA

my yoga path

How did my yoga practice go today?

*Know that when you lose
yourself, you will reach the
beloved.*

ANSARI OF HERAT

my yoga path

How did my yoga practice go today?

my yoga path

How did my yoga practice go today?

*Relaxation is when you start
to really enter the heart of
yoga.*

CYBÈLE TOMLINSON,
SIMPLE YOGA

my yoga path

How did my yoga practice go today?

check in

Use this page for general explorations of yourself and your yoga practice.

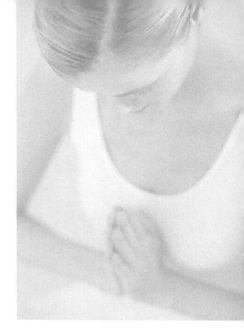

chapter four

the breathing
practices

We can live for weeks without food and days without water, but only a few minutes without oxygen. Our life itself is measured from our first breath to our last. Still, most of us don't give breathing a passing thought except when we have a head cold or visit that friend who lives in a fifth-floor walk-up.

In yoga, we learn that the breath is the bridge from body to mind, from outer concerns to inner peace. Breathing is used during *asanas* to assist in reaching our personal best (usually, inhalation accompanies an upward- or backward-bending movement, exhalation a downward- or forward-bending move). *Pranayama* is also an important practice in its own right.

Pranayama brings under your control the normally automatic function of breathing in order to regulate the flow of *prana*, or life energy, throughout your system.

With the exception of trained singers, elite athletes, and yogis, most people are shallow breathers who seldom completely fill their lungs with air or fully exhale stale air and start fresh. Learning *pranayama* can help you use your lungs' full capacity for breath. The result is greater vitality, clearer eyes and skin, and a better functioning respiratory system.

(This may be the reason many people who take up yoga say they get fewer colds than they did before.)

Some basics of *pranayama* are:

* Sit cross-legged on the floor or on a cushion. As an alternative, you can kneel or sit in an accommodating chair. In any case, avoid rigidity, but keep your back straight enough that your lungs feel open and free to expand.

* In most yogic breathing exercises, the exhalation should be one-and-a-half to two times as long as the inhalation. If this doesn't feel natural at first, advance slowly. Count your breaths to keep track.

* *Pranayama* is more about guiding the breath than controlling it. Unless your teacher instructs you otherwise, allow your body to breathe of its own accord and gently usher your breath where you want it to go.

By regulating your breathing, you can increase the oxygenation of your entire system, improve circulation, relieve tension and anxiety, and increase concentration. Breathing practices can also regulate the flow of *prana* or life energy in your body; and slow, steady breathing is an essential component of meditation. In addition to formal *pranayama*, you can do a simple yoga breathing routine during the day when you need to calm down, energize yourself, or clear your mind before giving a presentation or dealing with a problem.

The simplest practice is basic, three-part, deep breathing (*deergha swasam*). To do this, you inhale by extending first your abdomen, then your diaphragm, and finally your chest; and follow by exhaling slowly and fully, drawing your abdomen in as if to push out the last vestiges of stale air. Doing even three of these inhalation-exhalations has been shown to slightly lower blood pressure and steady brain wave patterns.

Most importantly, whenever you do a breathing practice—and whenever it crosses your mind during the day—observe the point of stillness between each inhalation and exhalation. This is a tiny meditative moment. When you momentarily focus on it during *pranayama*—and at other times as well—you gently train your mind to focus and, even in the midst of past memories and future plans, become acutely aware of the present.

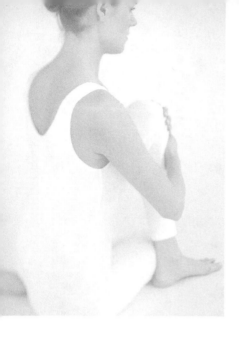

writing prompts

Let these suggestions spur your writing.
Don't feel the need to respond to all of them;
just write about the ones that speak to your heart.

1. Yoga is like a four-legged stool—postures, breathing, relaxation, and meditation—and each "leg" is of equal value. How much value does *pranayama* have in your personal practice? What benefits have you gained from it? What benefits do you expect?

2. It may not be possible in daily life to take a break from a board meeting to stand on your head, but you can pay attention to your breathing—thus the yogi's saying, "Breathe first. Act later." Make a list of times and places during your typical day when you might turn within and do some simple breathing practices.

3. Now write about the kinds of situations that you are likely to experience that would benefit from a bit of before-the-fact breathing. (Examples might be dealing with employers/employees, going for interviews or auditions, confrontations with difficult people, etc.)

4. How do you understand the underlying life force that the yogis call *prana*? How does knowledge of this invisible life force help you in your practical, everyday life?

my breath

In the box titled "I breathe in," list qualities you would like to attain. Under "I breathe out," list attributes you want to get rid of. During your next yoga practice, refer to this list and incorporate its affirmation into your practice: "I breathe in patience, I breathe out hurry," or "I breathe in courage, I breathe out fear."

I breathe in . . .	*I breathe out . . .*

*What lies behind us and
what lies before us are tiny
matters compared to what
lies within us.*

RALPH WALDO EMERSON

my yoga path

How did my yoga practice go today?

my yoga path

How did my yoga practice go today?

When you hold the breath,
you hold the soul.

B.K.S. IYENGAR

my yoga path

How did my yoga practice go today?

*The mind is connected with
the life force indwelling in
all beings. Like a bird tied to
a string: so is the mind.*

YOGA SHIKHA UPANISHAD

my yoga path

How did my yoga practice go today?

my yoga path

How did my yoga practice go today?

*All consciousness is
essentially one.*

FRITJOF CAPRA

my yoga path

How did my yoga practice go today?

*And the Lord God formed
man of the dust of the
ground, and breathed into
his nostrils the breath of life;
and man became a living
soul.*

GENESIS 2:7

my yoga path

How did my yoga practice go today?

check in

Use this page for general explorations of yourself and your yoga practice.

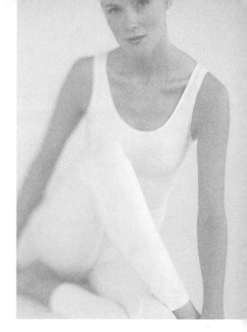

chapter five

meditation

When a yoga teacher first told me that meditation would do me good, I had two thoughts in rapid succession—both terrifying. First was, "I'll get bored." Second: "I'll miss something." But accepting my teacher's conviction that, in seeking out yoga, I was a ripe candidate for meditation, too, I started meditating. Sometimes I was bored, but I lived through it, gaining some patience in the process. And I don't think I've ever missed anything during meditation except a few phone calls I could return later.

We live in a glittery world with lots to attract our attention. Those of us who find the notion of meditation least appealing—we who are especially fond of action, momentum, excitement, and adrenaline—have an even greater need for this quieting practice than those calm people we've never understood much. We devotees of the high life tend to approach yoga class with the attitude, "I'll do the exercise part, but I'll leave before we have to just sit there or, heaven forbid, *chant*."

Like it or not, however, yogis both ancient and modern insist that the *raison d'être* of hatha yoga is to prepare the body for meditation, a practice that can still the thoughts, awaken the intuition, and lead to peace of mind and freedom of spirit. Even when meditation is done without the other aspects of yoga, independent medical research has shown that it improves physical and mental functioning. Regular meditators have been found to suffer less chronic disease and take fewer sick days. They even rank as "younger" in physiological age than nonmeditators.

Meditation is simply the act of bringing your awareness to a single point. That point might be the image of a holy personage, the light of a candle, the breath going in and out of your nostrils, or a *mantra*, a sound vibration. The most widely known *mantra* is *Om*, the Sanskrit word that is said to be the primordial sound, the sacred "Word" that brought all creation into being.

Whatever technique you choose, meditation is the quintessence of simplicity. It requires no equipment, only the willingness to persist, to return repeatedly to the point of focus. In meditation, you sit. Thoughts come. They're enticing. Interesting. Fascinating. But you don't go with them. You bring your awareness back to the image or the breath or the *mantra*.

Sometimes meditation has immediate rewards. You walk away after the practice feeling more peaceful or more positive than you did before you started, or you get some flash of intuition you can use in a practical situation. Much of the time, however, you won't feel anything. That doesn't mean nothing is happening. Even at these times, you're learning to become more focused. You're gaining control over the "monkey mind" that likes to swing from branch to branch, from concept to idea to memory to yearning. And at times you even touch the state that yoga refers to as "pure being," "field of consciousness," or "bliss"—the ultimate reality beyond the realm of day-to-day concerns.

Many serious meditators make time to practice in both the morning and the late afternoon or evening. If you can only meditate once a day, most people find that the best time is in the morning, after a shower and before breakfast, following *asanas* and *pranayama* if you're able.

The position most amenable to meditation is the same as that for *pranayama*: sitting comfortably upright on the floor or a cushion or in a straight-backed chair. The lotus posture (*padmasana*) is the classic meditation pose. This pose takes more hip flexibility than most Westerners have since we've sat in chairs since we were babies. Work up to it slowly. The ideal meditation posture for you today is the one in which you're most comfortable.

Once you're seated, start to watch your inhalations and exhalations, not controlling them in any way, simply watching. Then bring to mind your image or your *mantra* if you're using one, and gently bring your awareness back to that focus for the ten or twenty minutes you've set aside for meditation. Come back to the hustle-bustle world slowly. Writing in your journal is one way to accomplish this gentle return. If your religious faith calls for daily devotions, this is a good time to include them, because you are fully awake, fully relaxed, and open to inspiration.

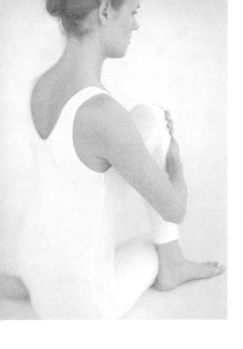

writing prompts

Let these suggestions spur your writing.
Don't feel the need to respond to all of them;
just write about the ones that speak to your heart.

1. Meditation can sometimes be boring, yet yogis have said that boredom can be the highest state of receptivity. Do a written rethink on the concept of boredom. What's positive about it? What does it have to teach you? How can you be less afraid of it?

2. Meditation, like yoga, is a discipline. Draw up for yourself a "positive report card" on how disciplined you are in various areas of your life—yoga practice, meditation, eating well, taking care of yourself, and meeting the responsibilities that are unique to your situation. Grade yourself honestly but kindly. Then write simple, doable ways to improve.

3. A man I knew gave up meditating. Some time later, he became angry and yelled at his wife. Although she had never meditated herself, she told him: "I liked you better when you meditated." He took it up again. If you have been meditating a while, what differences do you notice in yourself? What differences do you notice in your relationships?

4. Sometimes we get insights during meditation that are worth remembering. Write these in this journal. Even when you don't come away from meditation with a gem of wisdom, some meditation periods just feel especially good. Write about these, too.

my meditation

Give yourself a word-association test. Write down the following words and phrases, followed by the first thought that comes to mind when you do so.

meditation _____

contemplation _____

prayer _____

sitting _____

silence _____

quiet time _____

alone _____

doing nothing _____

breathing _____

waiting _____

being with my thoughts _____

taking time for myself _____

Are there any patterns or surprises in your thoughts? If so, write about what you've learned about yourself. Either way, commit to meditating every day for a month—even just five minutes a day if that's all the time you want to give it. At the end of thirty days, take this quiz again and see how your answers have changed.

From intuition, one knows everything.

THE YOGA SUTRAS OF PATANJALI

my yoga path

How did my yoga practice go today?

my yoga path

How did my yoga practice go today?

*I want to know God's
thoughts . . . the rest are
details.*

ALBERT EINSTEIN

my yoga path

How did my yoga practice go today?

my yoga path

How did my yoga practice go today?

*Listen to your own Self. If
you listen to that Self within,
then you find the Truth.*

KABIR

my yoga path

How did my yoga practice go today?

my yoga path

How did my yoga practice go today?

my yoga path

How did my yoga practice go today?

*You need not leave your
room. Remain sitting at your
table and listen. . . . The
world will freely give itself
over to you to be unmasked.*

Franz Kafka

*Even so large as the universe
outside is the universe within
the lotus of the heart.*

CHANDOGYA UPANISHAD

my yoga path

How did my yoga practice go today?

check in

Use this page for general explorations of yourself and your yoga practice.

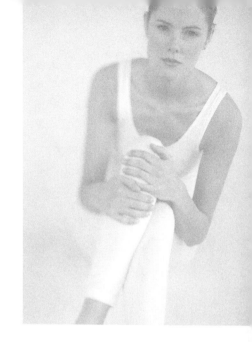

chapter six

diet

You may have noticed it already. If not, it's sure to happen:
the yoga student's nutritional revelation. You'll be tending to
the business of grocery shopping or ordering from a menu,
and it will hit you: "I'm eating better than I used to, and I
didn't even realize I was doing it."

Virtually all students find themselves eating healthier
foods after they've been doing yoga for a while. The yogic
explanation for this is that doing *asanas*, *pranayama*, and
meditation changes you at a cellular level. Foods that are
greasy, chemically preserved, or excessively sweet simply stop
looking good.

Beyond this gradual leaning toward more natural,
healthful foods, yoga teachings themselves include a detailed
philosophy of diet that categorizes foods in three classifica-
tions called *gunas*. They are: *tamasic*, or inert; *rajasic*, stimu-
lating; and *sattvic*, balancing.

Tamasic foods include anything stale or tasteless, left-
overs of more than a day, alcoholic drinks, chemical-laden
processed foods, aged cheeses, and anything deep-fried. Eating
these is believed to cause fatigue, laziness, and depression and
makes it easier to give in to the desires of the lower nature.

Rajasic foods are the stimulants: meats and eggs, salty or highly spiced dishes, refined sugar desserts and soft drinks, and beverages containing caffeine. These can provide a temporary energy boost, but it's an artificial energy that can lead to a letdown later.

Sattvic foods comprise the bulk of the yogic diet. In this category are whole grains, fresh fruits, raw or lightly cooked vegetables, nuts, beans, high-quality dairy products, and raw honey. Yoga teaches that a diet based on these foods leads to high-level health, a sharp mind, and a contented spirit.

The traditional yogic diet is vegetarian. This is both because most *sattvic* foods come from the plant kingdom and because the yogic tenet of *ahimsa*, nonharming, precludes all killing, even that of animals for food. If a vegetarian diet is attractive to you, it can be both health promoting and delicious. It is also believed to aid one's progress in yoga, but it is certainly not a requirement. Even some of the highest profile yoga teachers in the West today are not vegetarian. As in all other aspects of this practice and philosophy, you're free to take what fits for now and discard what doesn't.

In yoga, study and exploration are always encouraged. If you're interested in learning more about a vegetarian diet, contact The Vegetarian Resource Group (www.vrg.org), Physicians Committee for Responsible Medicine (www.prcm.org), or the North American Vegetarian Society (www.navs-online.org).

The overweening yogic attitude toward eating is moderation. "Even nectar," the yogis say, "becomes poison when eaten too much." This outlook reflects yoga's overall view of life and health: Eat enough but not too much. Sleep well but don't sleep late. Walk and dance and labor, but do not exhaust yourself. Enjoy every moment of life on earth, but know all the while that you live in eternity.

writing prompts

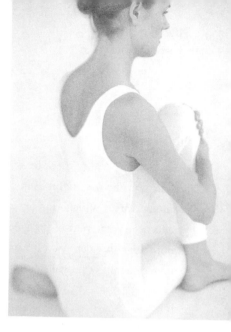

Let these suggestions spur your writing.
Don't feel the need to respond to all of them;
just write about the ones that speak to your heart.

1. Are you attracted to the idea of nourishing yourself in a more yogic fashion? What steps could you take to do this? Is there one step you're willing to commit to right now? How will you implement this change?

2. Has your diet changed since you started doing yoga? Do you feel differently about certain foods?

3. A vegetarian diet is one of the more controversial of yoga's suggestions. Write your feelings about the choice some people make to live without meat. Do you think it's wise? Are you interested but cautious? If so, what concerns you? Where will you go to learn more?

4. Is eating moderately difficult for you? Do you overeat or undereat? Do you go on weight-loss diets? How do you think yoga might help with this? What else might you look into to help you develop a healthier relationship with food?

my diet

Do a dietary reality check by writing down everything you eat and drink for three days on this chart. Put the *tamasic* foods in column one, the *rajasic* foods in column two, and *sattvic* foods in column three. Which kind of food predominates? Are you surprised? Does your personality reflect the yogic view of the type of food you're eating? In other words, do you find yourself more sluggish when you eat *tamasic* foods, more agitated when you eat a lot of *rajasic* foods, or more centered when your diet is primarily *sattvic*?

	TAMASIC	RAJASIC	SATTVIC
day one			
day two			
day three			

The simplest meals can be extraordinarily satisfying if they are prepared and served with care and with the intention to provide pleasure as well as sustenance.

ANDREW WEIL, M.D.,
EATING WELL FOR OPTIMUM HEALTH

my yoga path

How did my yoga practice go today?

my yoga path

How did my yoga practice go today?

*Because there is one bread,
we who are many are one
body, for we all partake of
the one loaf.*

I Corinthians 10:16-17

my yoga path

How did my yoga practice go today?

*Foods that promote life,
mental strength, vitality,
cheerfulness, and a loving
nature . . . are agreeable to
the sattva-natured person.*

THE BHAGAVAD GITA

*Our lives are not in the lap
of the gods, but in the lap of
our cooks.*

LIN YUTANG

my yoga path

How did my yoga practice go today?

my yoga path

How did my yoga practice go today?

my yoga path

How did my yoga practice go today?

I am oppressed with the dread of living forever. This is the only disadvantage to vegetarianism.

GEORGE BERNARD SHAW

check in

Use this page for general explorations of yourself and your yoga practice.

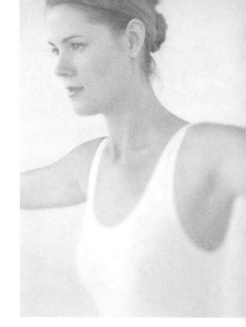

chapter seven

the ethical
precepts

As individuals, we may have strong spiritual beliefs, but our culture frowns on letting these strongly affect our dealings in the *real* world. Things were quite different in ancient India, where yoga developed. There, the touchstone of reality was the spiritual world, and life on earth was seen as a mere reflection, described by the Sanskrit word *maya*, illusion.

Believing that development of the soul was the purpose of living in a body, yoga's early teachers would only take on prospective students after they had mastered yoga's ethical precepts. It's different in the twenty-first century West. Usually only serious students who stay with yoga and study its principles outside class learn the ethical precepts at all. That's why these principles are discussed at the end of this book instead of the beginning. Even so, they form a firm foundation for a yogic way of life.

First of the ethical precepts are the *yamas* (disciplines). They are:

Ahimsa, or nonviolence—to avoid harming another being, through thought, word, or deed.

Satya, truthfulness—to speak the truth to others and face the truth in ourselves.

Asteya, nonstealing—to refrain from taking what is not ours and to acquire only those possessions that truly enrich our lives.

Brahmacharya, moral conduct regarding sex—to develop standards for ourselves in this area and live up to those standards.

Aparigraha, noncoveting—to keep any greediness in check and not lose ourselves to our desires.

The second set of ethical precepts are the *niyamas*, or restraints.

These are:

Shaucha, cleanliness—to keep our bodies clean, our thoughts pure, and our surroundings uplifting.

Santosa, contentment—accepting what we have with gratitude and finding peace within our current circumstances, even as we work to improve them.

Tapas, ardor—to do away with obstacles to our personal and spiritual growth.

Svadhyaya, self-knowledge—constant striving to know the truth about who we are in every sense.

Ishvara pranidhana, devotion to a Higher Power—for religious people, this means commitment to that religion and its teachings. For yoga students who are not religious, it is simply a humble acceptance of human limitations and an openness to the existence of something greater than human intellect and human power.

According to tradition, staying true to the *yamas* and *niyamas* clears the path to progress in yoga. Without its ethical underpinnings, yoga could be seen as little more than a combination of calisthenics and concentration. With them, yoga promises a way of life based on principles of conduct that honor the self and others. Following these tenets leads to a life that is rich, fulfilling, and ripe with promise.

Although you will benefit from yoga at whatever level of involvement you choose to have, delving deeply into its philosophy and practice will ground you firmly in the yogic way of life. Central to the yogic world view is that everything is connected to everything else. For this reason, no action we take and no choice we make is unimportant. Enlarging our ethical awareness doesn't just make us better people; it makes the world a better place.

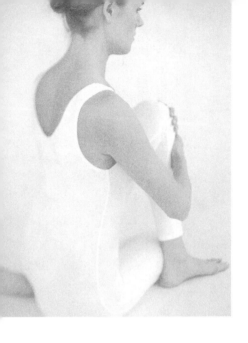

writing prompts

Let these suggestions spur your writing.
Don't feel the need to respond to all of them;
just write about the ones that speak to your heart.

1. On a first reading, which of the five *niyamas* (disciplines) jumps out at you or seems most important? List ten ways in which you might practice that observance more effectively in your daily life.

2. Of the *yamas* and *niyamas*, is there one that irritates or offends you or one that simply doesn't seem to apply to your life? Write about this precept. Explore what might be in it for you. See if there is a way to rethink the concept so it better fits your life and your view of the world.

3. Think of some difficulty, even a minor one, that you're experiencing with another human being. Write about how the focused practice of one or two of the *yamas* might improve your dealings with this person.

4. Create a "Yogi Unawares" award to give (in your journal, at least) to someone you know who beautifully embodies several of these principles. State what qualifies this person to be a yogi unawares. Include how his or her ethical values have made your life better.

5. Write about moral precepts in general. Should we have them, or should people be free to come up with their own? If one person adopts an ethical principle, should he expect others to hold to the same principle?

6. What has been your experience in dealing with the beliefs of others? How have you been able to honor your own ethical standards and still respect people who have different ones?

my yoga life

Write a brief paragraph on how each *yama* and *niyama* fits into your life. Review your responses every few months. If you want, make a copy of this page before you fill it in, and write fresh responses when you feel it's necessary.

Yamas

Ahimsa _____

_____

_____

Satya _____

_____

_____

Asteya_____

_____

_____

Brahmacharya_____

_____

_____

Aparigraha _____

_____

_____

Niyamas

Shaucha _____

_____

_____

Santosa _____

_____

_____

Tapas _____

_____

_____

Svadhyaya _____

_____

_____

Ishvara pranidhana _____

_____

_____

*Nobility of character
manifests itself at loopholes
when it is not provided with
large doors.*

Mary Wilkins Freeman

my yoga path

How did my yoga practice go today?

*If you have made up your
mind to find joy within
yourself, sooner or later you
shall find it.*

PARAMAHANSA YOGANANDA

my yoga path

How did my yoga practice go today?

my yoga path

How did my yoga practice go today?

If people speak ill of you,
live so that no one will
believe them.

PLATO

my yoga path

How did my yoga practice go today?

*Engage yourself in good
deeds, good company, and
good thoughts. Be good,
honest, and well-behaved.*

SRI SATYA SAI BABA

my yoga path

How did my yoga practice go today?

my yoga path

How did my yoga practice go today?

*What do we live for, if not
to make life easier for one
another?*

T.S. ELIOT

check in

Use this page for general explorations of yourself and your yoga practice.

Desikachar, T.K.V. *The Heart of Yoga: Developing a Personal Practice* (Rochester, VT: Inner Traditions, 1999).

Feuerstein, Georg, and Stephan Bodian, with the staff of *Yoga Journal. Living Yoga: A Comprehensive Guide for Daily Life* (Los Angeles: Jeremy P. Tarcher, 1993).

Monro, Dr. Robin, Dr. R. Nagarathna, and Dr. H.R. Nagendra. *Yoga for Common Ailments* (New York: Fireside, 1990).

Prabhavananda, Swami, and Christopher Isherwood. *How to Know God: The Yoga Aphorisms of Patanjali* (Hollywood: Vedanta Press and Bookshop, 1996).

Satchidananda, Sri Swami. *Integral Yoga Hatha* (Buckingham, VA: Integral Yoga Distribution, 1998).

Sivananda Yoga Vedanta Center. *Yoga Mind & Body* (New York: DK Publishing, Inc., 1998).

Tomlinson, Cybèle. *Simple Yoga* (Berkeley: Conari Press, 2000).

for further reading